Gratitude Journal

MAVEN PRESS

First published in Australia in 2024
by Maven Press
Roleystone WA 6111

NATIONAL LIBRARY OF AUSTRALIA

A catalogue record for this work is available from the National Library of Australia

National Library of Australia Catalogue-in-Publication

data: Gratitude Journal: Maven Press

ISBN: 978-0-6456356-9-0

(Paperback)

Gratitude

Introduction

Welcome to a journey towards cultivating joy, resilience and mindfulness through the power of gratitude.
This journal is more than just pages; it's a sanctuary for reflection and appreciation, a space where the ordinary transforms into the extraordinary.
Each entry invites you to explore the richness of your experiences, encouraging a mindful pause to acknowledge the blessings, big or small, that weave through the tapestry of your life.
Let these pages be a beacon of positivity, a compass guiding you to the heart of gratitude.
As you embark on this transformative journey, may your reflections spark waves of gratitude, shaping a life abundant with joy, connection and mindful awareness.

Gratitude

Gratitude

Date:

How do I feel today?

What did I do well today?

What am I feeling gratitude for?

3 positive things going forward today

Reflection

Be thankful for ...

Gratitude

Gratitude

Gratitude

Gratitude

Gratitude

Gratitude

Date:

How do I feel today?

What am I feeling gratitude for?

3 positive things going forward today

Be thankful for ...

What did I do well today?

Reflection

Gratitude

Gratitude

Gratitude

Gratitude

Gratitude

Gratitude

Date:

How do I feel today?

What am I feeling gratitude for?

3 positive things going forward today

Be thankful for ...

What did I do well today?

Reflection

Gratitude

Gratitude

Gratitude

Gratitude

Gratitude

Gratitude

Date:

How do I feel today?

What am I feeling gratitude for?

3 positive things going forward today

Be thankful for ...

What did I do well today?

Reflection

Gratitude

Gratitude

Gratitude

Gratitude

Gratitude

Gratitude

Date:

How do I feel today?

What am I feeling gratitude for?

3 positive things going forward today

Be thankful for ...

What did I do well today?

Reflection

Gratitude

Gratitude

Gratitude

Gratitude

Gratitude

Gratitude

Date:

How do I feel today?

What did I do well today?

What am I feeling gratitude for?

3 positive things going forward today

Reflection

Be thankful for ...

Gratitude

Gratitude

Gratitude

Gratitude

Gratitude

Gratitude

Date:

How do I feel today?

What did I do well today?

What am I feeling gratitude for?

3 positive things going forward today

Reflection

Be thankful for ...

Gratitude

Gratitude

Gratitude

Gratitude

Gratitude

Gratitude

Date:

How do I feel today?

What did I do well today?

What am I feeling gratitude for?

3 positive things going forward today

Reflection

Be thankful for ...

Gratitude

Gratitude

Gratitude

Gratitude

Gratitude

Gratitude

Date:

How do I feel today?

What am I feeling gratitude for?

3 positive things going forward today

Be thankful for ...

What did I do well today?

Reflection

Gratitude

Gratitude

Gratitude

Gratitude

Gratitude

Gratitude

Date:

How do I feel today?

What am I feeling gratitude for?

3 positive things going forward today

Be thankful for ...

What did I do well today?

Reflection

Gratitude

Gratitude

Gratitude

Gratitude

Gratitude

Gratitude

Date:

How do I feel today?

What did I do well today?

What am I feeling gratitude for?

3 positive things going forward today

Reflection

Be thankful for ...

Gratitude

Gratitude

Gratitude

Gratitude

Gratitude

Gratitude

Date:

How do I feel today?

What am I feeling gratitude for?

3 positive things going forward today

Be thankful for ...

What did I do well today?

Reflection

Gratitude

Gratitude

Gratitude

Gratitude

Gratitude

Gratitude

Date:

How do I feel today?

What am I feeling gratitude for?

3 positive things going forward today

Be thankful for ...

What did I do well today?

Reflection

Gratitude

Gratitude

Gratitude

Gratitude

Gratitude

Gratitude

Date:

How do I feel today?

What am I feeling gratitude for?

3 positive things going forward today

Be thankful for ...

What did I do well today?

Reflection

Gratitude

Gratitude

Gratitude

Gratitude

Gratitude

Gratitude

Date:

How do I feel today?

What am I feeling gratitude for?

3 positive things going forward today

Be thankful for ...

What did I do well today?

Reflection

Gratitude

Gratitude

Gratitude

Gratitude

Gratitude

Gratitude

Date:

How do I feel today?

What am I feeling gratitude for?

3 positive things going forward today

Be thankful for ...

What did I do well today?

Reflection

Gratitude

Gratitude

Gratitude

Gratitude

Gratitude

Gratitude

Date:

How do I feel today?

What am I feeling gratitude for?

3 positive things going forward today

Be thankful for ...

What did I do well today?

Reflection

Gratitude

Gratitude

Gratitude

Gratitude

Gratitude

Gratitude

Date:

How do I feel today?

What did I do well today?

What am I feeling gratitude for?

3 positive things going forward today

Reflection

Be thankful for ...

Gratitude

Gratitude

Gratitude

Gratitude

Gratitude

Gratitude

Date:

How do I feel today?

What am I feeling gratitude for?

3 positive things going forward today

Be thankful for ...

What did I do well today?

Reflection

Gratitude

Gratitude

Gratitude

Gratitude

Gratitude

Gratitude

Date:

How do I feel today?

What am I feeling gratitude for?

3 positive things going forward today

Be thankful for ...

What did I do well today?

Reflection

Gratitude

Gratitude

Gratitude

Gratitude

Gratitude

Gratitude

Date:

How do I feel today?

What am I feeling gratitude for?

3 positive things going forward today

Be thankful for ...

What did I do well today?

Reflection

Gratitude

Gratitude

Gratitude

Gratitude

Gratitude

Gratitude

Date:

How do I feel today?

What am I feeling gratitude for?

3 positive things going forward today

Be thankful for ...

What did I do well today?

Reflection

Gratitude

Gratitude

Gratitude

Gratitude

Gratitude

Gratitude

Date:

How do I feel today?

What did I do well today?

What am I feeling gratitude for?

3 positive things going forward today

Reflection

Be thankful for ...

Gratitude

Gratitude

Gratitude

Gratitude

Gratitude

Gratitude

Date:

How do I feel today?

What am I feeling gratitude for?

3 positive things going forward today

Be thankful for ...

What did I do well today?

Reflection

Gratitude

Gratitude

Gratitude

Gratitude

Gratitude

Gratitude

Date:

How do I feel today?

What did I do well today?

What am I feeling gratitude for?

3 positive things going forward today

Reflection

Be thankful for ...

Gratitude

Gratitude

Gratitude

Gratitude

Gratitude

Gratitude

Date:

How do I feel today?

What am I feeling gratitude for?

3 positive things going forward today

Be thankful for ...

What did I do well today?

Reflection

Gratitude

Gratitude

Gratitude

Gratitude

Gratitude

Gratitude

Date:

How do I feel today?

What did I do well today?

What am I feeling gratitude for?

3 positive things going forward today

Reflection

Be thankful for ...

Gratitude

Gratitude

Gratitude

Gratitude

Gratitude

Gratitude

Date:

How do I feel today?

What did I do well today?

What am I feeling gratitude for?

3 positive things going forward today

Reflection

Be thankful for ...

Gratitude

Gratitude

Gratitude

Gratitude

Gratitude

Gratitude

Date:

How do I feel today?

What am I feeling gratitude for?

3 positive things going forward today

Be thankful for ...

What did I do well today?

Reflection

Gratitude

Gratitude

Gratitude

Gratitude

Gratitude

Gratitude

Date:

How do I feel today?

What am I feeling gratitude for?

3 positive things going forward today

Be thankful for ...

What did I do well today?

Reflection

Gratitude

Gratitude

Gratitude

Gratitude

Gratitude

Gratitude

Date:

How do I feel today?

What am I feeling gratitude for?

3 positive things going forward today

Be thankful for ...

What did I do well today?

Reflection

Gratitude

Gratitude

Gratitude

Gratitude

Gratitude

Gratitude

Date:

How do I feel today?

What am I feeling gratitude for?

3 positive things going forward today

Be thankful for ...

What did I do well today?

Reflection

Gratitude

Gratitude

Gratitude

Gratitude

Gratitude

Gratitude

Gratitude

Gratitude

www.ingramcontent.com/pod-product-compliance
Lightning Source LLC
Chambersburg PA
CBHW080359030426
42334CB00024B/2926
* 9 7 8 0 6 4 5 6 3 5 6 9 0 *